This book b... ...

A Pocketbc
for
Safer IV Therapy

A Pocketbook
for
Safer IV Therapy

(Drugs, Giving Sets and Infusion Pumps)

Martin Pickstone, PhD, BSc, Dip Mat Sc, DMS
Honorary Research Fellow
Imperial College School of Medicine
London

Scitech Educational

Acknowledgements

We are indebted to all the enthusiastic people from the following organisations who have contributed ideas and information for this book: Alaris Medical Systems, Arcomedical Infusion Ltd, Baxter Healthcare Ltd, Derbyshire Royal Infirmary NHS Trust, Greycoat Publishing, The Hammersmith Hospitals NHS Trust, Imperial College School of Medicine, Medical Devices Agency, Royal College of Nursing, Scitech technical authors, SIMS Graseby Limited, Newcastle-upon-Tyne Hospitals NHS Trust and University of Derby.

Distributed by Scitech-DIOL

© Scitech Educational Ltd 1999

Reprinted 1999 with additions

ISBN 0 948672 32 3

The views expressed are those of the authors and do not necessarily reflect those of Scitech Educational Ltd.

Published by

Scitech Educational Limited, Margate, Kent CT9 1TE, United Kingdom
Tel: +44 (0) 1843 231494
Fax: +44 (0) 1843 231485
http://www.scitechdiol.co.uk

Printed in Great Britain by Alpha Publishing

Preface

In the United Kingdom, one of the most serious types of medication error is that which involves the use of infusion pumps. One serious incident a month is reported: half of these incidents end in a patient death[a]. Furthermore the number of serious but not fatal incidents is understated because NHS Trusts are only under a statutory duty to report unexpected patient deaths. Studies of industrial accidents have shown that for every serious or fatal injury, there are thousands of unsafe practices and conditions that do not cause injury[b]. The origin of this book was an investigation of the number of types of unsafe clinical practices that are associated with the use of infusion pumps[c]. One hundred and two types were identified. So the proposition that each serious infusion incident rests on a bed of many thousands of unsafe practices is very plausible. The number of patient injuries can be reduced only by training clinical staff to use infusion systems (pumps and associated equipment) competently; for competence improves both the safety and quality of clinical practice.

What is competence? We know instinctively that to drive any motor car safely in all road, traffic and weather conditions is competent driving. The competent driver uses skills to cope safely with many different kinds of challenging circumstances. These skills (known as transferable skills) are a combination of background knowledge (The 'Highway Code'), specific skills to control the vehicle and driving experience. This book is intended to be the equivalent of the motorist's 'Highway Code' for clinical staff who use infusion systems to administer intravenous drug therapy. The book is based on the preparatory workbook for 'Finger-on-the-Button' (a system of training to use infusion systems competently) that has been developed by Scitech Educational for the Imperial College School of Medicine.

(a) The average rate of incidents reported to the Medical Devices Agency between November 1994 and June 1997.

(b) Heinrich H W, Petersen D, Roose N. *Industrial Accident Prevention, a Safety Management Approach.* London: McGraw Hill, 1980, 20 - 73.

(c) Investigations undertaken between 1994 & 1996 for 'Finger-on-the-Button' (a system of training to use infusion systems competently) that has been developed by Scitech Educational Limited for the Imperial College School of Medicine.

In this book intravenous therapy is treated as a three-stage process that determines the sequence and content of the chapters. First the drug dose is calculated - Chapter 1. Then the drug is made up as a solution - Chapter 2. Finally the infusion system (the pump and associated equipment) is selected to meet the patient's need and the safety requirements of the intravenous therapy - Chapter 3.

Martin Pickstone, London

CONTENTS

Chapter 1

Drug Calculations for IV Therapy

In this chapter:

1.1 Weights
1.2 Concentrations
1.3 Calculating concentrations
1.4 Dosage
1.5 Infusions

Chapter overview

At the heart of infusion systems are infusion pumps - the devices which deliver the required dose rate and dose of the drug to the patient. They must be carefully and properly set up. However, pumps have to be loaded with the correct quantity of drug, and sometimes you may have to load a mixture of drugs. This means that to set up an infusion system properly, you need to know exactly what the system is going to supply. So first of all, we will discuss weights, concentrations and dosages of drugs.

We will cover:

■ Grams, milligrams, micrograms and nanograms and the relationships between them
■ How to work out the strengths of solutions
■ How to work out the proper dosage (and infusion rates) for administration to a patient.

If you are quite confident you know all there is to know and can handle the calculations without difficulty, then try the revision questions at the end.

1.1 WEIGHTS

The amounts of a drug you give to patients are incredibly small. Usually you talk about grams, milligrams, micrograms, sometimes even nanograms but have you ever stopped to think just how small these are? You weigh about 60 kilograms and 'kilo' means 1000. This means you weigh about 60000 grams. A milligram is one thousandth of a gram or one sixty millionth of your body weight. A microgram is a thousand times smaller than that so obviously, you have to be absolutely certain of the differences between these names.

1 kilogram	= 1000 grams
1 gram	= 1000 milligrams
1 milligram	= 1000 micrograms
1 microgram	= 1000 nanograms

To change	from	to	do this
	kilograms	grams	multiply by 1000
	grams	milligrams	multiply by 1000
	milligrams	micrograms	multiply by 1000
	micrograms	nanograms	multiply by 1000
	nanograms	micrograms	divide by 1000
	micrograms	milligrams	divide by 1000
	milligrams	grams	divide by 1000
	grams	kilograms	divide by 1000

Examples:

500 milligrams	= 500/1000	= 0.5 grams
1250 micrograms	= 1250/1000	= 1.25 milligrams
0.25 grams	= 0.25 x 1000	= 250 milligrams
0.05 milligrams	= 0.05 x 1000	= 50 micrograms

If you abbreviate these weights, make sure you use the correct terms, and especially remember to use small (lower case) letters;

kilogram	kg
gram	g
milligram	mg
microgram	microgram
nanogram	ng

Many Trusts' drug policies state that abbreviations should not be used to reduce the risk of errors occurring.

1.2 CONCENTRATIONS

Concentrations arise when you have substances dissolved in a solvent, usually but not always, water. They are a measure of how much is dissolved in a certain amount of solution so you always have to refer to them as 'amount of substance per amount of solution'. You can't refer to them as just an amount of substance alone because that would be meaningless unless you say how much water or other solvent there is as well. So far as these calculations are concerned, it doesn't matter if the solvent is water or saline or 5% glucose - what is important is that you know exactly how much of a substance is present in a given amount of solution.

To begin with, a few words about volumes. There are still a lot of different terms in common use - pints of milk or beer, litres of petrol or even, occasionally, gallons but the standard unit in hospital use, as elsewhere, is the litre, abbreviated to 'l' or the millilitre (ml) equal to one thousandth of a litre. If you need to get a feel for these amounts in terms of, say, milk bottles, a litre is a bit less than two pints.

In the case of concentrations, we've got four different ways to say what we mean.

- Percentage concentrations when the dissolved substance is measured in grams and the solvent is fixed at 100 millilitres (ml). These are referred to as '% w/v'.

A 1% w/v solution means 1 gram dissolved in 100 ml
A 20% w/v solution means 20 g dissolved in 100 ml
A 55% w/v solution means 55 g in 100 ml

and so on.

■ Percentage concentration when the dissolved substance is measured in millilitres and the solvent is fixed at 100 ml. These are referred to as '% v/v' and are used when a solution is made by dissolving one liquid in another.

A 1% v/v solution means 1 ml dissolved in 100 ml of liquid
A 40% v/v solution means 40 ml in 100 ml of liquid

and so on.

■ Weight or volume ratios. Again very similar but now we don't have to base the measurement on 100 ml of liquid. We can use any amount (weight or volume) dissolved in any volume so long as we state the amounts. Quite often, the amount of solution specified is one litre.

5 grams per litre simply means what it says - 5 grams of solid contained in 1 litre of liquid
25 g/500 ml means 25 g of solid dissolved in 500 ml of liquid
1 in 1000 means 1 g in 1000 ml (1 g/litre or 1 mg/ml)

■ Molar solutions. These will be familiar if you did chemistry at school or college, but if you didn't or if you've forgotten about them, the following is a brief explanation. (As with the calculations, you may be able to skip the next few paragraphs: they are intended for you if you didn't study chemistry.)

The 'mole' is a unit of mass used in science and it relates to the molecular weight (to use the old term) or 'relative molecular mass', abbreviated to RMM, of a compound. It also refers to the relative atomic mass, (or RAM) of an element.

A molar solution of a drug is the relative molecular mass of the drug, expressed in grams, in 1 litre of solvent.

All elements (and there are 92 of them that occur naturally, from hydrogen up to uranium) exist as atoms. Atoms are so minute that their individual weights are immeasurably small. To solve this problem, the mass of each element's atom is measured relative to a reference which is now Carbon 12. The table shows the relative atomic masses (RAMs) of a selection of elements (rounded to the nearest whole number).

Element	RAM
Hydrogen	1
Carbon	12 *
Oxygen	16
Sodium	23

* Reference atom

The Periodic Table found in every chemistry text book lists the RAM of all 92 elements.

When it comes to compounds (like water, alcohol, glucose or drugs with complex chemical structures such as adrenaline), the molecules are made up of atoms chemically joined together. Each molecule has a mass and its relative molecular mass (RMM) is worked out by adding up the RAMs of all the atoms in the molecule.

A molar solution of any compound is the relative molecular mass dissolved in 1 litre of solvent.

So water, with a formula H_2O, has a RMM of

$$2 \times 1 + 1 \times 16 = 18$$

Ethanol, formula C_2H_5OH is made up of two carbon atoms, six hydrogen atoms and one oxygen atom so its RMM is

$$2 \times 12 + 6 \times 1 + 1 \times 16 = 46$$

1.3   CALCULATING CONCENTRATIONS

1.3.1   Changing ratios to % solutions

% solutions are always based on 100 ml of solvent. Here are three examples:

Example 1

> 5 g/l = 5 g/1000 ml
> divide by 10 to base it on 100 ml
>   = 0.5 g/100 ml
>   = 0.5% w/v

Example 2

> 25 g/500 ml
> divide by 5 to base it on 100 ml
> = 5 g/100 ml
> = 5% w/v

Example 3

> 50 ml in 250 ml water
> divide by 2.5 to base it on 100
> = 20 ml in 100ml water
> = 20% v/v

If your mathematics is a little rusty for changing ratios to % solutions, perhaps an easier way to remember is:

'divide by what you have and multiply by what you want'.

In Example 1, we've got 1000 ml but we need to base it on 100 ml for a % solution; so divide the 5 g by 1000 (what you have) and multiply the answer by 100 (what you want). In Example 2, we've got 500 ml but we want to base it on 100 ml so we divide by 500 and multiply the answer by 100. In Example 3, divide by 250 and multiply by 100.

1.3.2   Changing % solutions to ratios

It's just as straightforward to go the other way.

Example 4

To change a 35% w/v solution to g/l:

> 35% w/v = 35 g in 100 ml
> divide by what you have (100 ml)
>   = 0.35 g in 1 ml
> multiply by what you want (1 litre or 1000 ml)
>   = 350 g/l

Example 5

To change 10% v/v solution to ml/l:

> 10% v/v = 10 ml in 100 ml of solution
>   = 0.1 ml in 1 ml of solution
>   = 100 ml/litre

1.4 DOSAGE

These calculations often come down to finding out how much of a given strength solution must be used to ensure the patient receives the correct amount of a drug and we can use the same approach as we used above for the concentration calculations.

Example 6

Suppose you have a solution labelled '200 g/l' and you have to administer only 5g of the dissolved material. How much of the solution should you give?

Well, you have 200 g in 1 litre of the solution but you only want 5 g.

So divide 1 litre or 1000 ml by 200 (what you have) which gives you the number of ml that contains 1 g.

   1000 ml/200 g = 5 ml/g

So 5 g is contained in 5 x 5 ml, i.e. 25 ml.

So you would administer 25 ml of the solution.

Calculate the volume of solution that contains 1 g (or 1 mg for example). Then multiply the volume by the number of grams (or mg for example) you need to administer.

Example 7

For your next patient, you have to give 50 mg of a drug using a solution labelled 10% w/v.

How much of the solution do you give?

> 10% w/v = 10 g in 100 ml (watch out for g and mg!)
> = 10000 mg in 100 ml

Divide by what you've got (10000 mg) and multiply by what you want (50 mg)

> = 1 mg in 0.01 ml
> = 5 mg in 0.5 ml

So you would administer 0.5 ml.

Example 8

You have been told to make up 250 ml of a 20% w/v solution of a certain compound in water. What weight of solid and volume of water would you use?

> 20% w/v = 20 g in 100 ml

Divide 20 g by what you have (100 ml) and multiply by what you want (250 ml).

> 20/100 ml x 250
> = 0.2 g in 1 ml x 250
> = 50 g in 250 ml

You would dissolve 50 g of the compound in 250 ml of water.

Don't be confused by a concentration such as '1 g of lignocaine in 500 ml glucose 5%'. This simply means that the solvent is not water but 5% glucose. Any calculation is exactly the same as the ones above. For example, 1 g of lignocaine in 500 ml glucose 5% is the same as 0.2 g in 100 ml; in other words, a 0.2% w/v solution in 5% glucose.

1.5 INFUSIONS

We're concerned with giving drugs to patients over an extended period of time, perhaps several hours. Obviously the infusion pump will be used for this but someone still has to key in the right settings on the pump so that it delivers the correct amount over the correct period of time.

Now you also have to deal with rates of addition and that means bringing time into the calculation. Later on, we'll meet infusion calculations that depend on the patient's body weight or size as well as time but for the moment, we'll just concentrate on time alone.

Example 9

Lignocaine is to be administered at a rate of 1 mg/min using a solution containing 1 gram of lignocaine in 500 ml glucose 5%. What is the infusion rate in ml/min?

> 1 g lignocaine in 500 ml
> = 1000 mg in 500 ml

What we have is 1000 mg in 500 ml and what we want is 1 mg. So divide 500 ml by 1000 and multiply by 1 to give the volume that contains 1 mg.

> 500/1000 x 1 = 0.5 ml

and if we infuse the patient at a rate of 0.5 ml/min, the patient will be receiving 1 mg/min of lignocaine; just what the doctor ordered!

Example 10

You have an isoprenaline infusion prepared containing 5 mg in 500 ml glucose 5%. What is the infusion rate to ensure the patient receives 2 micrograms/min of isoprenaline?

> 5 mg in 500 ml
> = 5000 micrograms in 500 ml

You've got 5000 micrograms and you want 2 micrograms - so divide by 5000 and multiply by 2.

> = 1 microgram in 0.1 ml
> = 2 micrograms in 0.2 ml

and the correct infusion rate is 0.2 ml/min.

If you want to set the pump to give this infusion rate per second or per hour instead of per minute, all we have to do is remember there are 60 seconds in a minute and 60 min (or 3600 s) in an hour:

> 0.2 ml/min
> = 0.2 ml/60 seconds

What we've got is 60 s, what we want is 1 s. So divide by 60 and multiply by 1.

> = 0.0033 ml/s

and to change it to ml/hour:

> 0.2 ml/min (you have 1 min and we want 60 min so divide by 1 and multiply by 60)
> = 12 ml/hr

Now we'll bring body weight or body size into the calculation. The patient's weight is easy to find but for body size (measured as surface area, in m^2) you'll need special tables or nomograms.

Example 11

You have a dopamine solution containing 800 mg in 500 ml glucose 5%. The patient is a 70 kg man and he is to have 10 micrograms (mcg) of dopamine/kg/min. How many ml/hour should be set on the pump?

First, you'll need to work out what this particular patient needs. He is to have 10 micrograms/kg/min and he weighs 70 kg so his dosage must be 10 x 70 = 700 micrograms/min. The rest is exactly the same as all the other calculations:

    800 mg in 500 ml
    = 800,000 micrograms in 500 ml

You have 800,000 micrograms, you want 700 micrograms. So divide by 800,000 and multiply by 700:

    = 1 microgram in 0.000625 ml
    = 700 micrograms in 0.4375 ml

and the patient needs 0.4375 ml/min of the solution to ensure that 10 micrograms/min for every kg of body weight is received.

Finally, we have to set the pump in ml/hour, so:

    0.4375 ml/min, multiplied by 60
    = 26.25 ml/hour.

Example 12

An infusion solution is labelled 10% w/v and the drug has to be infused at a rate of 200 mg/min. What is the infusion rate in ml/min and also in ml/hour?

$$10\% \text{ w/v} = 10 \text{ g in } 100 \text{ ml}$$
$$= 10{,}000 \text{ mg in } 100 \text{ ml}$$
$$= 200 \text{ mg in } \frac{100}{10{,}000} \times 200 \text{ ml} = 200 \text{ mg in } 2 \text{ ml}$$

$$\therefore \text{ Rate } = 2 \text{ ml/min or } 120 \text{ ml/hour}$$

Infusion rates based on body size are handled in precisely the same way. For example, the dose might be 80 mg/m^2 and the patient's surface area (found using tables or nomograms) is 1.84 m^2.

In this case, the patient needs a total dose of 80 x 1.84 = 147.2 mg. If this has to be infused at a certain rate you should by now be able to work out the pump setting without difficulty.

1.5.1   Drip rate calculations

Drip sets deliver carefully controlled amounts of liquid in droplets at a set rate.

A standard solution set will administer 20 drops per ml of clear fluid (in other words, each drop should have a volume of one twentieth of a millilitre).

A blood giving set will administer 15 drops per ml of blood (20 drops per ml of clear fluid).

Some burette sets will administer 60 drops per ml.

It is important to double check the number of drops per ml delivered by the set on the outer packaging as these may vary slightly between products.

To see how to work out the drip rate to ensure the patient receives the correct amount of a drug at the correct rate, let's do a similar problem to one we've already done - only instead of adding the drug by pump, we're going to add it by drip.

Example 13

A drug is to be given to an 80 kg man at a rate of 10 micrograms/kg/min. The solution to be used contains 160 mg in 100 ml glucose 5%. What is the drip rate using a standard solution set delivering 20 drops/ml of clear fluid?

As before, we'll first use the patient's weight to work out the particular dose for him.

He needs 10 micrograms/kg/min and he weighs 80 kg. Therefore he needs 10 x 80 = 800 micrograms/min.

Now look at the solution we have to use:

160 mg in 100 ml of glucose 5%
= 160000 micrograms in 100 ml

We have 160000 micrograms and we want 800 micrograms. So divide by 160000 and multiply by 800:

= 1 microgram in 0.000625 ml
= 800 micrograms in 800 x 0.000625 ml
= 800 micrograms in 0.5 ml

If we were using the pump, we would set it to 0.5 ml/min. But we're not - we're using a standard solution set which delivers uniformly sized drops and there are 20 drops to each ml of fluid. We only need 0.5 ml/min so that means 10 drops/min.

There is a little formula to calculate the required drip rate (once you've worked out the volume needed) which you might find helpful:

$$\text{Number of drops per minute} = \frac{\substack{\textit{Volume} \\ \textit{needed (ml)}} \times \substack{\textit{Number of drops/ml} \\ \textit{delivered by the set}}}{\textit{Duration of the infusion (minutes)}}$$

Example 14

A drug is to be administered using a standard solution set at a rate of 50 mg/m²/min to a patient whose surface area is 1.6 m². The stock solution is 4% w/v. What drip rate should be used?

The patient requires   50 x 1.6   = 80 mg/min

4% w/v   = 4 g in 100 ml
= 4000 mg in 100 ml

We have 4000 mg; we want 80 mg, so we divide by 4000 and multiply by 80:

= 1 mg in 0.025 ml
= 80 mg in 2 ml

The patient needs 2 ml/min of the solution and using the formula:

$$\textit{Number of drops per minute} = \frac{\substack{\textit{Volume} \\ \textit{needed (ml)}} \times \substack{\textit{Number of drops/ml} \\ \textit{delivered by the set}}}{\textit{Duration of the infusion (minutes)}}$$

The standard solution delivers 20 drops per ml of clear fluid, so:

$$\textit{Number of drops/minute} = \frac{2 \text{ ml} \times 20}{1 \text{ minute}}$$

$$= 40 \text{ drops/minute}$$

The way to make these calculations easier is to do them one step at a time. Don't try to rush them - just lay them out, line by line, and get into the routine. Speed can come later once you are confident and can work out any problem without difficulty.

There are two other important areas you should know, namely 'Divided doses' and how to find and use the 'Displacement Value' of a drug.

1.5.2   Divided doses

Sometimes the dose is quoted as a 'total daily dose' or TDD which has to be given in divided doses, usually three or four times a day.

It's important to distinguish between the total daily dose and individual doses otherwise you might give the patient three or four times the specified dose!

Example 15

'Ibuprofen, 1200 mg daily in three divided doses' means 1200 mg given in three equal doses - in other words, 1200/3 = 400 mg every 8 hours for a total of 1200 mg over the whole day. 'Day', of course, means 24 hours so that 'four divided doses' means dividing the total daily dose into four equal parts and administering each part every 6 hours. 'Every 4 hours' would mean dividing the total daily dose into 24/4 = 6 equal amounts. 'Cefuroxime I.V. 2.5 g daily in two divided doses' would mean giving 1.25 g every 12 hours.

1.5.3   Displacement values

Some drugs, especially antibiotics, have been freeze-dried. They are in solid form in the vial and need to be reconstituted before they can be administered. This is done by adding a known value of fluid to the vial.

However, these powders displace a certain amount of fluid - known as the 'Displacement value' or sometimes 'Displacement Volume' of the drug and these amounts must be taken into account when part vials are being used. Unless this is done, you could make serious errors in dosage, especially when the doses are small, for example for babies.

You'll find displacement values in the relevant data sheets or in paediatric dosage books, and the best way to explain how to use them is to work through a few examples. What you must remember is that the displacement value and the amount of fluid you add together make up the total amount of fluid in the vial.

Example 16

To give a dose of 125 mg amoxycillin from a 250 mg vial. The displacement value for amoxycillin 250 mg is 0.2 ml.

If you add 4.8 ml of fluid you will then have a total of 5 ml in the vial (the displacement value, 0.2 ml, plus the 4.8 ml you added).

So you have 250 mg in 5 ml. However, you only want 125 mg so you would administer half the solution, or 2.5 ml.

Example 17

Cefotaxime is to be given to a baby at a dose of 50 mg/kg, 12 hourly. The baby weighs 3.6 kg. The Cefotaxime is in a 500 mg vial and its displacement value, for a 500 mg vial, is 0.2 ml.

Dosage required = 50 x 3.6 = 180 mg, 12 hourly
Displacement value for Cefotaxime 500 mg = 0.2 ml
Add 1.8 ml water to give a total of 1.8 + 0.2 ml = 2 ml
You now have 500 mg in 2 ml

You need to give 180 mg, so divide by 500 and multiply by 180

= 180 mg in (2 ÷ 500) x 180 = 0.72 ml

and you administer 0.72 ml, 12 hourly.

Example 18

*Dosage required: 50 mg/kg from a 500 mg vial. Patient is a child weighing 8
kg. Drug has a displacement value of 0.3 ml. You need to reconstitute the drug
as a solution of 5 ml. What volume should be administered?*

Dosage required = 500 x 8 = 400 mg
Displacement value of the drug, 500 mg = 0.3 ml
Add 4.7 ml water making a total of 4.7 + 0.3 = 5 ml in the vial

You have 500 mg in 5 ml

400 mg is dissolved in (5 ÷ 500) x 400 = 4 ml

You administer 4 ml.

We can work out the difference if you do not allow for the displacement value.

In Example 17, suppose we had added 5 ml to the vial. We would then have
drawn up 2.5 ml as before. But, in fact, there would be 5.2 ml of fluid: in other
words, 250 mg in 5.2 ml. But the actual dose in 5 ml is:

(250 ÷ 5.2) x 5 = 240.4 mg in 5 ml

Now if we draw up 2.5 ml, we only have drawn up 120.2 mg of the drug - not
125 mg. Nearly 5 mg less!

In Example 18, if we had added 2 ml to the vial, it would actually have contained 2.2 ml of water.

We would have 500 mg in 2.2 ml and if we still administered 0.72ml, we would only have drawn up:

$(500 \div 2.2) \times 0.72 = 164$ mg of Cefotaxime

16 mg less than we should have given!

1.6 REVISION QUESTIONS

(1) Express 75 g/500 ml solution as a % solution. Will it be w/v or v/v?

(2) Change 200 g/l to a % w/v solution.

(3) Express a 45% w/v solution as g/l.

(4) 250 ml of solution contains 1750 mg of a drug. What is this as a % w/v solution?

(5) How would you make up a 500 ml of 5% w/v glucose solution?

(6) The dosage required is 100 mg of a drug using a solution labelled 5% w/v. What volume would you administer?

(7) You have to administer a drug which is only available as a 75% v/v solution. You would administer 3 ml of a 100% v/v solution. How much would you administer of the 75% v/v solution to provide the same drug dose in 3 ml of 100% v/v solution?

(8) Lignocaine has to be infused at a rate of 150 mg/min using a 10% w/v solution of lignocaine in glucose 5%. What is the pump setting? State it in ml/min and also in ml/hour.

(9) You have a solution labelled 5% w/v and you have to infuse the drug at a rate of 100 mg/min. What is the infusion rate in ml/hour?

(10) Nitroprusside is to be given to a 60 kg man at a rate of 2 µg/kg/min. The infusion solution contains 50 mg in 100 ml glucose 5%. What is the correct pump setting in ml/hour?

(11) A drug has to be infused at a rate of 800 microgram/min using a solution labelled 0.5 g/l. What is the infusion rate in ml/min and ml/hour?

(12) A drug is to be administered using a standard solution set at a rate of 75 mg/m²/min to a patient having a surface area of 1.7 m². The solution strength is 5% w/v. What drip rate should be set, in drops/min and also in drops/hour?

(13) Infusion required is 1 mg/kg/min to a patient weighing 60 kg. Using a standard solution set and a solution labelled 5% w/v, what is the drip rate in drops/min?

(14) What must you *always* check before using a drip set?

(15) 500 ml saline 0.9% infusion over 8 hours. What is the infusion rate per hour? What is the rate per minute?

(16) Using Example 18, how big an error do you make if you ignore the displacement value of the drug and add 5 ml of water instead of 4.7 ml but still administer 4 ml to the patient?

Chapter 2

Drug Interactions in IV Therapy

In this chapter:

2.1   Chemical breakdown of drugs
2.1   Precipitation
2.3   Interaction with plastic components

Chapter overview

In the last chapter, we discussed how to calculate the amount of drug to be given. IV therapy often requires several drugs to be administered simultaneously. We now need to consider how they interact with each other. To add to the complexity of the situation, the plastic tubing we use to deliver drugs can interfere with the drugs' rate of delivery.

We all know that ordinary, everyday materials eventually change, either because of the way we use them or, apparently, just by time alone. For example, iron rusts, copper turns green, milk turns sour, and so on. Everything we use is a chemical and chemicals react under the right (or wrong) conditions to form new substances. Drugs are chemicals, so it ought not to come as a surprise if under certain conditions they react or precipitate out of solution.

When this happens, the drug might be rendered useless, or not as strong as the dosage suggests; or it might even be converted into a form that may be hazardous to the patient. So you have to be aware of the possibilities and know the basic steps you can take to prevent or minimize these changes.

2.1 CHEMICAL BREAKDOWN OF DRUGS

First of all, we'll take a broad look at what can cause drugs to react and so cause the problem of becoming less potent or unusable. For the moment, we'll only consider single drugs - later, we'll also consider drugs used in combination and the particular problems that might cause.

The problems can arise from three main areas; either:

- By chemical attack or the influence of light or
- The drug might be caused to precipitate out of solution and so block tubing and cannulae or
- Because the drug is incompatible with the plastic tubing used in the administration set or solution bag.

Let's take a look at each of these in turn. Chemical breakdown of a single drug can happen in any of several ways including:

- Hydrolysis
- Oxidation or reduction
- Photolysis or light degradation.

2.1.1 Degradation by water (hydrolysis)

Intravenous administration requires the drug to be dissolved either in water or in a water-based liquid like glucose or saline. However, water may react with the drugs that are dissolved in it by a chemical process called hydrolysis. Fortunately, degradation by hydrolysis is not often a significant problem in clinical practice. Hydrolysis is likely to occur with drugs that need to be reconstituted before use because they are relatively unstable in the presence of water.

The acidity or alkalinity of the solution can also promote hydrolysis. The term pH (always a small p, big H) is the measure of acidity or alkalinity of a solution. pH uses a numerical scale ranging from 0-14 with 7, the half-way point, being a completely neutral solution.

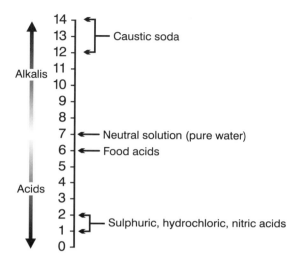

Fig. 1 pH scale

Pure water is neutral, having a pH of 7, while acids have a pH of below 7 and alkaline solutions (or basic solutions as they are sometimes called) have a pH of between 7 and 14. A strong acid (like sulphuric, hydrochloric or nitric) has a pH of around 1 or 2; whereas the so-called food acids (like citric) have a pH of about 6. On the other side of the scale, strong alkalis like sodium hydroxide (caustic soda) have a pH of about 12-14 and a weak alkali typically has a pH of about 8-9.

Hydrolysis is often accelerated by inappropriate pH changes. In other words, a diluent is added (or a second drug, if a combination is being used) which causes the solution to become more acidic (lower pH) or more alkaline (higher pH). Even the small difference in pH between saline 0.9% or glucose 5% injections, for example, can dramatically affect the stability of some drugs, such as ampicillin, amphotericin or erythromycin.

There are two other important points about pH. The first is that even materials which are not obviously acids or alkalis can have acidic or alkaline (basic) characteristics, and they can therefore have a pH value on the acid or alkaline side of neutral. For example, glucose 5% has a pH of approximately 4.0-4.2, depending on the manufacturer. The second is that pH changes can often be controlled by adding a 'buffer solution'. The chemistry of 'buffers' is quite complex but they work by chemically mopping up excess acidity or alkalinity. As a result, the pH of a buffered solution will stay fairly constant despite the addition of either acidic or alkaline solutions.

However, not many drugs are so unstable around the pH range of 5 - 7.5 that they lose significant activity under normal clinical conditions. What degradation might occur can usually be minimised or even prevented over a 24 hour period by using the recommended diluent. For example, the use of glucose solution to reconstitute ampicillin would decrease the stability to one half in 24 hours. At pH 5.5 or below, erythromycin is unstable with 10% decomposition occurring in 8-9 hours; if glucose is used as the diluent (for example for sodium-restricted patients), it may be necessary to add a buffer to prevent too great a change in pH.

Temperature can also affect the rate at which hydrolysis occurs and here the general rule is, the higher the temperature the faster the reaction. But as with pH effects, this is not usually a serious problem under normal clinical conditions.

2.1.2   Degradation by oxidation/reduction

Most chemicals react with oxygen, some faster than others and drugs are no exception. Some, like adrenaline, dopamine and ascorbic acid, can react quite readily and, like hydrolysis, the higher the temperature, the faster the reaction.

Oxygen is the vital component of the air we breathe, but oxidation of drugs by air is not a severe problem because air contains only 21% of oxygen. Most drugs are packaged and stored under airtight conditions as a precautionary measure. The degradation of drug solutions can eventually occur over a period of time but under normal conditions, oxidation is not usually a severe problem.

Some drugs (dopamine and noradrenaline in particular) might undergo a slight colour change (usually pink) and this is evidence of oxidation. A slight discoloration might represent minimal levels of degradation but does not necessarily indicate a safety hazard. However, discoloured solutions are *not* recommended for use.

Some drugs react with chemical reducing agents that remove oxygen from the drug molecules to produce a different compound. Thiamine is particularly prone to attack by reducing agents and the effect is worse at higher temperatures.

2.1.3   Degradation by light (photolysis)

We all know about the effects of sunlight - photosynthesis, for example, or causing sun-burn. These all involve chemical reactions, so we shouldn't be surprised that certain drugs can be affected by light as well.

The main problem for those drugs which are affected is natural daylight or (to be more precise) the UV radiation present in daylight. Drugs prone to light-induced degradation include :

- ■   Frusemide
- ■   Ergotamine
- ■   Nitroprusside
- ■   Vitamins A and K
- ■   Dacarbazine.

Amphotericin B is also susceptible and the manufacturers recommend light protection for aqueous solutions although several reports indicate that for short term exposure of 8-24 hours, little difference in potency is observed between light-protected and light-exposed solutions. However, longer periods of exposure may result in unacceptable potency loss.

With one important exception, fluorescent light is safe because it does not emit UV radiation. The one exception is nitroprusside which is very sensitive and degrades rapidly both by fluorescent light and natural daylight - or even a UV lamp. Therefore light protection of the infusion bag and administration set is essential for nitroprusside.

Vitamins A and K can also undergo significant degradation. In general, the best advice for all drug administrations is to protect them from strong daylight or sunlight - and be even more careful with nitroprusside.

2.2   PRECIPITATION

A drug meant for injection or infusion is obviously supposed to stay in solution. How else otherwise would you get it to flow through tubing and catheters into the body? If for any reason the drug precipitates (comes out of solution) it will be pharmacologically inactive and may be hazardous to the patient. A precipitate can block tubing, filters, cannulae or catheters and may, in theory, lead to coronary and pulmonary emboli if administered to the patient. Drug precipitation must therefore be avoided.

So what could cause the drug to precipitate? Well, mixing drugs that react with each other is an obvious possibility but for the moment, let's stay with single drug systems.

2.2.1   Precipitation and pH

Surprisingly many drugs are not very soluble in water when in their original chemical form; so they have to be converted into salts which are readily dissolved in water. There are two ways of doing this.

Some (the chemically acidic drugs) are converted into salts of the metals sodium or potassium. Others (chemically basic) are reacted with acids to form acid salts (hydrochloric, sulphate, nitrate, etc.).

Drug salts are water-soluble but are also sensitive to pH changes. If the pH changes as you make up a drug in solution, or dilute it or add another drug to it, then precipitation might occur.

The acidic drugs (which are converted into salts of sodium or potassium) generally have an alkaline pH in solution, the most alkaline having a pH greater than 9. Examples of drugs in solution that have a high pH (alkaline) are phenytoin, folic acid and most barbiturates. When these solutions are diluted in more water, saline or glucose solution, the pH decreases. If the pH falls too much and the water solubility of the drug in its original acid form is low, a precipitate may form.

Similarly, a typical basic drug (when formulated as an acid salt such as hydrochloric, sulphate or nitrate) forms an acidic solution (pH 3-5). Dilution of these salts raises the pH towards 7 and if the solubility of the original drug in its basic form is low, then a precipitate might form. Gentamicin is an example.

It's easy to see that dilution makes the solution either less acidic or less basic and so changes the pH of the solution much closer to the middle of the range. The drug then changes back to its original, relatively insoluble form and may well precipitate out of solution. As a general rule, the acidic drugs (the sodium or potassium salts in alkaline solution) are more likely to precipitate on dilution than the basic drugs.

There can be other causes. For example, if an alkaline solution - the sodium or potassium salt of an acid drug - is allowed to stand a long time in contact with air, it might absorb enough carbon dioxide from the air to lower its pH and so cause precipitation to occur. Carbon dioxide dissolves in water to form an acidic solution.

However, the more likely reason for precipitation is the mixing in the infusion container or the administration set of two drugs of very different pH, especially if one is acid and the other alkaline. One or both of the drugs might precipitate out simply because of the change in pH that we've already considered. Buffering might prevent this (remember, a buffered solution is one that doesn't change significantly in pH even if acid or alkali is added).

Sometimes the drug itself rather than a salt form can be used and then solubility is not affected by changes in pH. Insulin is one such example.

2.2.2   Precipitation and other dilution effects

Some drugs are so poorly soluble in water that they have to be dissolved or solubilized using co-solvents with water. Examples of these co-solvents are ethanol, polysorbates and propylene glycol. If the solution is then diluted with saline, for example, the co-solvents are further diluted and the drug may then precipitate.

If the solution is not diluted by much (for example, by only an equal volume of water) the concentration of co-solvent might still be high enough to keep the drug in solution. On the other hand, if the solution is very heavily diluted (say by adding 50 times as much water) there would then be enough water present to dissolve even a poorly soluble drug. It is between these extremes of dilution that a precipitate can form. Two common examples of drugs likely to precipitate on dilution are diazepam and digoxin but there are many more.

Now we shall move on to solutions that contain mixtures of drugs or other chemicals. We've already considered the risk of precipitation due to mixing two drugs of different pH. There are two other risks to be aware of.

2.2.3   Drug-drug co-precipitation

Drugs that have been converted into salts exist in solution as ions which are molecules that carry an electric charge. If one drug is positively charged and the other is negatively charged, then when the solutions are mixed, the ions will be attracted to (and react with) one another. A so-called 'ion pair' is formed which is insoluble and precipitates out of solution. Examples of drugs at risk of this kind of ion-pair interaction include:

- Gentamicin and heparin
- Frusemide and aminoglycosides.

These interactions must be avoided. A drug must never be allowed to mix with another drug to form an insoluble ion-pair that would then block up the administration line or cannula.

2.2.4   Formation of an insoluble salt

This problem occurs with the 'acid' drugs which are supplied as salts of sodium or potassium. You probably remember from chemistry lessons that all sodium and potassium salts are soluble which is precisely why these elements are used. But not all elements make the acid drugs soluble. In particular, metals like calcium, magnesium and iron form salts which are often insoluble. If calcium, magnesium or iron salts are allowed to mix with an acid drug, they can react to form an insoluble salt with the drug. In other words, the drug precipitates out.

Probably the most common example of a calcium-containing infusion is Hartman's Solution and this must not be mixed with an acid drug.

2.2.5   A question of time!

There is one final but important point about precipitation. The rate at which the precipitate forms depends on time: some precipitates may form almost immediately but in other cases, it may take several hours before the precipitate becomes visible. There are no simple rules but where precipitation is thought possible, the drug solution must be inspected carefully and frequently.

2.3   INTERACTION WITH PLASTIC COMPONENTS

Almost all containers, administration sets and components are made from plastics and unfortunately, a few drugs will bind to these plastics. This can obviously affect the rate of dose delivery and might even cause the rate to change with time.

There are three types of process that can occur and each can have a different effect on the drug delivery.

2.3.1   Interaction by adsorption

This is where the drug binds only to the surface of the plastic and does not penetrate any further. Adsorption doesn't happen with all drugs: in fact, only a very small number are affected. Adsorption reduces the concentration of the drug solution delivered to the patient and causes the dose delivered to change with time in an unexpected manner.

The initial effect is a rapid and substantial drug loss as the drug binds to the surfaces of containers and administration sets. The surfaces then become saturated and the concentration of drug in solution increases rapidly. Note that a solution that is administered intravenously is called an infusate. Figure 2 shows how the adsorption of insulin onto PVC affects the concentration of drug solution (infusate) over time.

The drugs most likely to be affected by adsorption are:

■   Insulin
■   Interferons.

Insulin will adsorb onto any plastic, especially PVC and also on to glass. To avoid or minimise the risk, insulin should not be added to the fluid container but should be given by syringe pump only at more than 1 unit/ml.

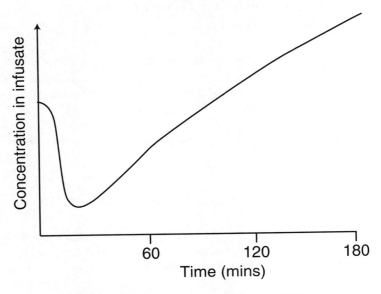

Fig. 2 Adsorption effects of insulin onto PVC

2.3.2 Interaction by absorption

This is where the drug actually migrates into the body of the plastic and is a more common occurrence than adsorption. Absorption is a slower process than adsorption and eventually, an equilibrium is established between the drug within the plastic and the drug in solution. The plastic becomes saturated with the drug and cannot accept any more. The drug concentration in the infusate is initially low but recovers more slowly than during adsorption.

PVC presents the biggest problem. PVC is made pliable and flexible by incorporating a 'plasticiser' during manufacture and this presents a particular problem for lipid-soluble drugs that diffuse from the solution into the plasticiser within the PVC.

The drugs most affected are:

- Diazepam
- Chlorpromazine
- Nimodipine
- Carmustine.

2.3.3   Interaction by permeation

In this case, the drug migrates through the plastic to the outer surface where it evaporates. Losses from permeation can be substantial and they continue all the way through the period of administration because the plastic never becomes saturated - see Figures 3 and 4. Again, PVC presents the biggest problem but nylon is also permeable to some drugs.

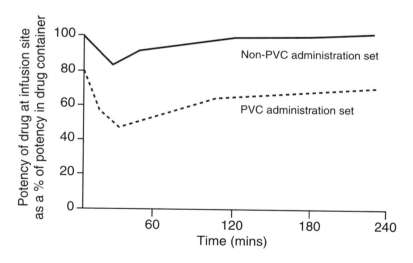

Fig. 3 The effect of permeation on the potency of chlormethiazole

The drugs most affected are:

- Nitrates
- GTN/ISDN
- Chlormethiazole.

Putting actual numbers on the magnitude of any drug loss due to binding with the surface is very difficult because so many factors are involved: drug concentration, flow rate, the surface area of the plastic, the type of plastic and the temperature. In most cases, the only solution is to avoid the plastic that allows the problem to occur (invariably PVC but also nylon) and change to polyethylene which does not absorb drugs.

There is an additional problem that can occur with PVC. The plasticiser added during manufacture to make it a flexible plastic can leach out into the drug solution. The effect is not usually important except for storage of all-in-one TPN regimens in PVC bags. Leaching from administration sets during the infusion is relatively small but it can occur from the rubber plungers of plastic syringes and may affect drug stability (for example, asparaginase).

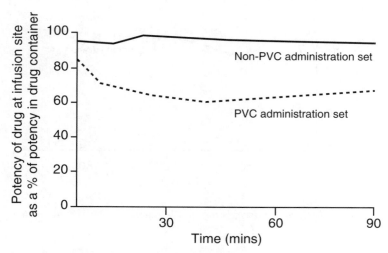

Fig. 4 The effect of permeation on the potency of isosorbide dinitrate

2.4   REVISION QUESTIONS

(1)   List THREE ways that a drug in solution for an infusion might be chemically broken down.

(2)   Explain, as concisely as you can, why simply diluting a drug in a solution bag might cause it to precipitate.

(3)   Name ONE drug that is especially sensitive to light.

(4)   Name THREE other drugs that are also light sensitive.

(5)   Why is ampicillin normally made up in saline 0.9% (sodium chloride solution) rather than glucose 5%?

(6)   Why might you need to be careful when diluting diazepam?

(7)   List TWO risks of mixing two drugs together.

(8)   Why should you be especially careful to check an infusion system frequently?

(9)   What is the difference between adsorption, absorption and permeation?

(10) Which plastic is most affected by these processes?

(11) Which plastic is least affected?

(12) Why must insulin be given by syringe pump and not added to the solution bag?

(13) Name TWO drugs in each case that are especially affected by (i) adsorption (ii) absorption and (iii) permeation.

(14) What might a pink coloration in noradrenaline suggest?

(15) Why should you not mix Hartman's solution with an acid drug?

Chapter 3

Drugs, Giving Sets and Infusion Devices for IV Therapy

In this chapter:

Chapter overview

Infusion pumps, giving sets and gravity drips are devices for automatically delivering the prescribed drug dose to the patient. They must be carefully and properly set up before use. The practical details of all the pumps that you will meet and the correct procedures that must be followed should be covered by training. This chapter aims to provide you with important background information; so we will be considering a number of issues around the pumps as well as information about the pumps themselves.

3.1 CONCENTRATIONS AND VOLUMES FOR INFUSIONS

The infusate or infusion fluid is a solution of one or more drugs dissolved in a liquid and the strength of the solution is measured in one of the ways considered earlier in this book. It might be % w/v or % v/v or, for example, 1 in 1000 - but whichever way is used it will always show the amount of drug in a given amount of liquid.

The solution might be concentrated or dilute. In other words, the drug might be dissolved in a small amount of liquid or, in a dilute solution, the same amount will be dissolved in a very much larger amount of liquid. So, to administer a given amount of a drug, you must know the concentration of the solution.

Example 19

To administer 1000 mg of a drug using a 50% w/v solution would require a volume of 2 ml but to administer the same amount using a 5% w/v solution would require 20 ml.

You can always work out the amount of drug administered by remembering the formula:

Amount of Drug = Concentration of Solution x *Volume*

where:

Drug concentration is expressed as the weight per unit volume of solution.

Alternatively, the volume of solution needed can be worked out:

$$Volume\ Needed = \frac{Amount\ of\ Drug}{Drug\ Concentration}$$

This is worked out as follows:

(1) 50% w/v solution means 50g in 100ml which is the same as 50,000mg in 100ml. So to administer 1000mg of the drug needs a volume given by:

$$\frac{Amount\ of\ Drug}{Drug\ Concentration} = \frac{1000\ mg}{50,000\ mg\ per\ 100\ ml}$$

$$= \frac{\cancel{1000}}{50,\cancel{000}} \times 100ml$$

$$= 2ml$$

(2) A 5% w/v solution means 5g in 100ml which is the same as 5000mg in 100ml. So to administer 1000mg needs a volume given by:

$$\frac{Amount\ of\ Drug}{Drug\ Concentration} = \frac{1000\ mg}{5000\ mg\ per\ 100\ ml}$$

$$= \frac{\cancel{1000}}{\cancel{5000}}$$

$$= 20\ ml$$

If you have any doubts at all, you should refer back to Chapter 1. The important point is that the same dose could be achieved by a small volume of highly concentrated solution and by a large volume of dilute solution.

3.2   ADMINISTRATION METHODS

There are three administration methods:

(1)   **A bolus/IV push**
This is usually given over three to five minutes.

(2)   **An intermittent infusion**
This is used as an alternative to bolus administration for regular dosing. Used where slower administration of a more dilute solution is required to avoid toxicity.
For example, vancomycin must be given at a maximum rate of 10 mg per minute to avoid red man syndrome.
For example, erythromycin must be diluted to at least 5 mg in 1 ml to reduce the risk of thrombophlebitis.

(3)   **Continuous infusion**
This term is given to infusions that are given continuously over at least 24 hours to achieve a controlled therapeutic response. The rate may either be variable or not. A drug that has a short half life or a narrow therapeutic window should be infused continuously. The half life of a drug is the time needed for the dose in the body to be halved and thus a drug with a short half life will be eliminated from the body quickly. In most cases, no drug will remain after a time interval of four half lives. For example, the half life of heparin is approximately one hour, so four hours after a bolus, none of the drug is left in the patient. Heparin is therefore infused continuously to maintain a stable dose and an unvarying therapeutic effect to treat thromboses.

Aminophylline has a narrow therapeutic window which means that there is a narrow range of drug concentrations in the plasma between which the drug exerts a therapeutic effect without toxicity. It is vital to maintain the drug concentration within this range for safety and effectiveness.

3.3 THE ADMINISTRATION SET

The components that make up administration sets are shown on the next two pages. Manufacturers can provide any combination of components but if your requirements are special, then the cost of bespoke manufacture for your Trust will be higher than that of standard items. The components shown will vary from manufacturer to manufacturer and so the drawings do not represent all variants. Volumetric pumps require a specific administration set that is recommended by the manufacturers.

Figure 5(a).
A.   Standard solution set.
B.   Standard blood set with 170 micron filter.
C.   Cannula for peripheral site. The cannula has a steel inner needle to puncture the vein and is then withdrawn. This cannula has an extension line of its own and a three way stopcock is also shown (see 'N' below).
D.   150 ml burette for neonatal infusions with a volumetric pump shown with an air inlet port E.
E.   Air inlet port, see above.
F.   Roller clamp for closing off any administration line.
G.   Silicone rubber insert in ordinary PVC tubing for use in infusions because this rubber does not distort or 'creep' when compressed by the volumetric pump mechanism. Silicone rubber improves the accuracy of the administration set for those pumps that use the *peristaltic pumping mechanism.*
H.   Pressure disc for measuring pressure in the administration set during an infusion. Used in sets for some volumetric and syringe pumps.
I.   'Y' connector for entry of another drug into the line.
J.   Spike for insertion into the fluid bag, shown with its own air inlet port.
K.   Luer lock with female and male screw fittings.

Figure 5(b)
L.   Narrow bore extension set for attachment to a syringe pump, shown with an in-line pressure-sensing disc.
M.   Four-way lumen for central venous site which can infuse four drugs separately each with its own lumen.
N.   Three-way stopcocks so that additional drugs can be infused into a lumen or a peripheral line. They do carry the risk of infection.
O.   Anti-siphon valve insert into a narrow bore extension set.

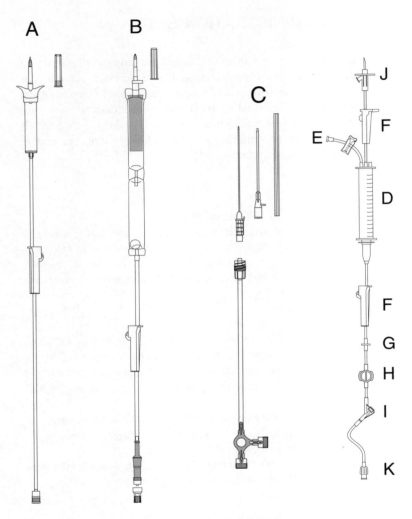

Fig. 5(a) Administration set components

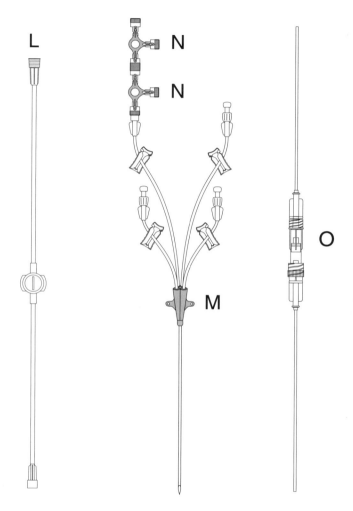

Fig. 5(b) Administration set components

3.4 DRUG ADMINISTRATION PROBLEMS WHEN USING INFUSION PUMPS

3.4.1 Air release from the fluid

There is no consensus of medical opinion about the risks associated with air entering the body during an infusion. Many people can tolerate the presence of air but too much air is lethal for all. However a proportion of the population has intracardiac circulation that can allow air and particles to travel from the left to the right side of the heart and thence into brain's circulatory system. Under some conditions, a bubble of air as small as 100 microlitres could constitute a hazard.

It may seem inexplicable and bizarre that gases dissolve in liquids just as sugar or salt dissolve in water. For example, undoing the cap of a bottle of lemonade releases gas, carbon dioxide, as pleasurable clouds of bubbles. The reason for the sudden burst of bubbles is that more of the gas dissolves in the lemonade under pressure. When the pressure is released and the bottle is left open to the atmosphere, a new lower level of carbon dioxide remains in solution which is why the lemonade then tastes 'flat'. However, the lemonade still contains carbon dioxide but not enough to flavour the drink.

Shaking a newly opened bottle is an explosive reminder that mechanical agitation of a liquid will also bring the gas out of solution. The reason why fizzy drinks remain drinkable is that bubbles only form slowly unless the bottle is either shaken or heated. Bubbles form at particular places on the inside of the container. These are called 'nucleation sites' and contain microscopically sharp irregularities and crevices upon which the bubbles can grow.

Air dissolves in IV fluids and drug solutions for the same reason that carbon dioxide dissolves in fizzy drinks. It comes out of solution in the same way too - as bubbles. The peristaltic and other mechanisms that volumetric pumps use, all mechanically agitate the infusate and can cause bubbles of excess air to form. However the manufacturers of fluids do exclude most of the dissolved air during the distillation and sterilising of water that is used to make solutions of saline and glucose.

Bubble detectors are incorporated into volumetric pumps as safety features but their clinical value has to be determined by clinicians and nurses in the context of the IV therapy and the condition of the patient. They work in two ways:

■   All individual bubbles that are greater than a minimum size are detected. The lower cut-off point can be adjusted in some models.
■   The total volume of all bubbles is measured and an alarm given when this volume has reached a set limit (which can be adjusted on some models).

3.4.2   Uncontrolled (free) flow

Uncontrolled emptying (free flow) can occur from gravity drips, volumetric pumps and syringe pumps. Free flow is dangerous, almost certainly causes an overdosage and can result in death.

Typical examples of when free flow can occur are as follows:

■   A roller clamp can be seen on all kinds of solution sets. The clamp is intended either to clamp or close the line completely, or to constrict flow in the line. The flow of drug solution will be uncontrolled if the clamp is left wide open. In this case the patient may suffer an overdose.
■   If the door of a volumetric pump is opened and the set removed, but the roller clamp is NOT closed, then uncontrolled flow will occur.

Volumetric pumps are used to administer large amounts of dilute solutions of drugs; and most modern volumetric pumps now have an anti-free flow device fitted to the set that prevents uncontrolled flow. *However, the roller clamp should still be closed as an instinctive safe habit.*

A drop detector is an extra safety device fitted to some volumetric pumps. The detector is attached to the drip chamber of the administration set and can indicate uncontrolled flow. When the infusion rate is set, the drop detector is then controlled by the pump's computer as to how many drops per minute correspond to the chosen rate. If the drop rate becomes larger than the expected value, then free flow is occurring. If the drop rate decreases, then the fluid bag is almost empty.

Uncontrolled flow from a syringe is called siphonage and there are two reasons for it:

(a) Gravity and
(b) Leakage of air into the syringe and administration set.

Siphonage can happen whether or not the syringe is fixed into a pump.

Free flow by gravity will always occur when the syringe exceeds a critical height above the infusion site - if either the barrel or the plunger is free to move. At this critical height, the head of fluid in the administration line and the syringe is just enough to overcome the venous pressure plus the friction in the plunger and the pressure drop in the administration line. Flow will stop only when the head of fluid is the same as the venous pressure. This critical height can be as low as 80 cm (30 inches) so in practice, the syringe is usually completely emptied.

Siphonage can be prevented by securely loading the syringe into the syringe pump. However, if the plunger is not engaged in the pump driver head, then it is free to move and at the critical height siphonage will occur. Also, if the plunger is engaged in the pump driver head but the barrel is loose, then the syringe may empty.

Siphonage can also occur by air leakage. This occurs more easily than by gravity because in this case, there is only the venous pressure to overcome. Usually, of course, the plunger has to move for the liquid to flow but if air enters, the syringe can empty without the plunger moving. The critical height, without the friction between plunger and barrel to overcome, can be as little as a few centimetres.

The time taken for the syringe to empty, whether by gravity or by air leakage, depends on the resistance to flow offered by both the administration line and the cannula. This resistance to flow, in any tube, is in turn controlled largely by the tube length and its internal diameter (also known as the 'bore'). A narrow tube offers more resistance than a wide one and similarly, the resistance of a long tube is greater than a short one. In the administration line, the resistance is due more to its length than its bore because it is both longer and wider than the cannula. In contrast, resistance to flow in the cannula is due more to its very small internal diameter.

In practice, a 50 ml syringe attached to a length of administration line with an internal diameter of 3 mm has been shown to empty by siphonage in less than one minute.

3.4.3 The importance of delivery and occlusion pressures

The pressure that is applied by the pump to achieve the desired flow rate has to overcome both the venous pressure and the resistance in the lines and filter (if fitted) and the intrinsic resitance of the fluid (the viscosity).

(1) Venous pressure

Flow into the vein will occur if the pressure at the tip of the catheter is slightly above the pressure in the surrounding vein. Typical venous pressures are:

- Adults, around 25 mm Hg to a maximum of 80 mm Hg
- Neonates, around 5 mm Hg.

(Hg is the chemical symbol for the liquid metal mercury and pressure is often measured in millimetres of mercury.)

(2) **Pressure due to line resistance**

There are two factors to be considered for line resistance - the bore and the line length. A wide bore tube needs a low velocity of flow to achieve a chosen volume flow rate (in ml/hour) – see Figure 6, Tube 1. The administration line is of fairly large bore, so its resistance is low. An in-line filter causes a resistance of about 10 mm Hg at 100 ml/hour, although all resistances vary with flow rate. The higher the flow rate, the higher the resistance to flow. The catheter, being of small bore, causes a significant resistance. (A narrow bore tube needs a high velocity flow rate to achieve the same flow rate as a larger bore tube – see Figure 6, Tube 2.)

So the rate of sliding or 'shear' between layers of liquid is low and resistance is low. The narrow bore Tube 2 needs a high velocity of flow to achieve the same volume rate as in Tube 1. The rate of sliding or shear between layers of liquid is high and the resistance is high.

Tube 1 - Wide bore causes low resistance

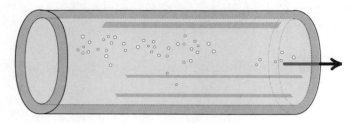

Tube 2 - Narrow bore causes high resistance

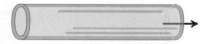

Fig. 6 Resistance to flow - bore of the tube

The length of the tubes causes variation in the resistance to flow. The greater the line length, the greater the resistance to flow – see Figure 7, Tubes 3 and 4. The velocities of flow are the same in both tubes. What differs is the areas of the layers of liquid in the tubes. The greater the length, the larger the areas of adjacent layers, and the more force is needed to slide the layers past one another.

Tube 3 - Short length causes low resistance

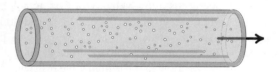

Tube 4 - Long length causes high resistance

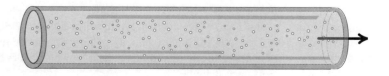

Fig. 7 Resistance to flow - length of the tube

(3) Pressure due to viscosity

The fluid itself, or (strictly) its viscosity, also causes resistance to flow. Viscosity is the internal friction of a liquid when it is on the move, caused by layers of liquid sliding past one another. The larger the molecules of the liquid, the more resistance they offer one another and the higher the viscosity. Figure 8 illustrates this showing a drug (pure – not in solution) with spherical molecules in a tube. Figure 8 also shows a liquid with smaller molecules having a lower viscosity. Most fluids used in medicine, however, have a viscosity similar to water and so the contribution of viscosity to resistance is the same in most IV therapies. The common exception is glucose solution.

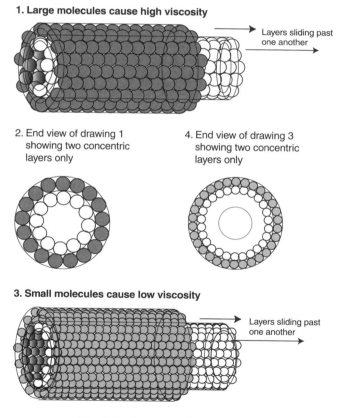

Fig. 8 Resistance to flow - viscosity

Example 20

How to calculate the maximum working pressure of a pump.

Imagine a 16G catheter 90 mm long. This will have a resistance of about 10 mm Hg at 100 ml/hour while the administration set will be much lower at about 1 mm Hg. Taking the maximum adult venous pressure of 80 mm Hg and allowing 10 mm Hg for an in-line filter, the total pressure to overcome will be:

$$10 + 1 + 80 + 10 = 101 \text{ mm Hg}$$

The pump will therefore have to achieve a maximum working pressure of about 120 mm Hg to maintain flow without alarming. Even allowing for other factors such as patient movement, the occlusion pressure need be set no higher than 220 mm Hg for the elimination of nuisance alarms during the infusion. For a neonatal infusion, the resistance to overcome is very much less.

---

(4) Occlusions

It is important that the vein must be patent during an infusion. If the vein is occluded, the patient will not receive the drug. The longer the occlusion occurs, the greater will be the pressure developed in the line because, of course, the pump will carry on pumping. Infusion pumps can generate high pressures if they are not controlled by appropriate pressure alarm levels. During the occlusion, the drug dose in the patient will not be maintained and so it will start to decrease which may be harmful. Leakage of the drug into the perivascular tissues (usually referred to as extravasation or tissuing) may also occur and this can be very dangerous.

The time to alarm will depend on the flow rate. If the rate is high, the pressure at which the pump alarms will be reached quickly. But if the rate is low, the pump will take a long time to reach the alarm pressure.

The setting of the occlusion alarm level is important because of the volume of stored bolus on release of the occlusion. For example, the back pressure when infusing a neonate at a flow of 1 ml/hour is unlikely to exceed 25 mm Hg. If the occlusion alarm pressure of the pump is set at, say, 50 mm Hg, then the pump will respond quickly to a total occlusion. A typical variable pressure pump would alarm in about three minutes under these conditions and the maximum stored bolus would be about 50 microlitres. On the other hand, if the pressure level was set at 300 mm Hg, the corresponding alarm time could be as long as 30 minutes with a stored bolus of about 0.4 ml. To release this into a vein could be dangerous.

3.4.4 Mechanical backlash

Syringe pumps suffer from 'mechanical backlash' which prevents the pump from immediately delivering the prescribed administration rate.

There are three causes of backlash:

(a) The syringe plunger is not tightly engaged in the pump driver head. Priming the syringe after loading the pump will always solve this problem.
(b) There is always some slack in the mechanism that can only be removed by starting the infusion. Some of the latest models eliminate the slack automatically.
(c) Friction in the syringe between the barrel and plunger can cause a jerky start to the emptying of the syringe. The extent of this will vary from syringe to syringe and also depend on the make.

If the infusion rate is very low, then the duration of the backlash is extended. The full therapeutic effect of the drug will then be delayed because the patient is receiving the dose more slowly than prescribed and this delay may be clinically significant.

All prescribed IV therapies assume that the preset rate is achieved instantly the pump is started.

3.4.5   Mechanical stability of the drip stand

The infusion device is usually fixed to a drip stand that has to be positioned somewhere close to the patient. In some cases, space may be restricted and accidents can happen when too many people (visitors, even overworked medical and nursing staff) need to be near the patient. Patients are encouraged to move around, often while receiving an infusion, so they have to push the stand when walking.

The drip stand that carries several pumps can be toppled over easily. Care must be taken to prevent overloading and mechanical instability.

3.4.6   Radio frequency interference

This is a serious and growing source of interference to critical care equipment arising mainly from the use of mobile phones and short-wave radios (as used by the emergency services, for example). Sparking in power cables, plugs and sockets that have been damaged by rough handling can also cause interference.

You may know that the use of mobile telephones, two-way radios and other electronic devices is banned on aircraft because the radio waves they emit can affect the aircraft's navigation and other equipment. They can have an equally serious effect on electromedical equipment including CTG monitors, infusion devices and external pacemakers.

The precise effects that mobile phones and short-wave radios have on equipment is always unpredictable. There are many different models of portable telephone and very many different types of electromedical equipment, each with its own level of susceptibility to interference. However, there is no way that the use of mobile phones will stop simply because they might interfere with medical equipment. They are here to stay so the only solution is to control their use within the hospital and especially in the vicinity of sensitive electromedical equipment.

The key factor is how close the source of interference (phone, radio, etc.) is to the medical device. The 'danger zone' around all devices, except for external pacemakers, is 1 metre for mobile phones and 2 metres for emergency service radios. For external pacemakers, the corresponding danger zones for these phones/radios are 4 and 26 metres respectively.

The distances mean that mobile telephones should not be used or left switched on, nor should two-way radios be used to transmit messages, in any of the following areas:

- In any clinical area.
- In any corridor, lift or room adjacent to a clinical area
- In any room or corridor that is either one or two floors above or below a clinical area
- In any courtyard, path or walkway outside the hospital which is within 10 metres of any clinical area.

Ambulatory patients with attached active equipment need to be accompanied by medical staff who are familiar with the equipment when entering the so-called 'safe' areas. Portering staff need to use their radios in the 'receive' mode as much as possible. The same applies to the emergency services (police, fire, etc.), particularly the fire service who may access any part of a building and transmit on short wave radios during a real or practice emergency. The only compromise to these rules is that security and all emergency staff should continue to use mobile phones/two-way radios with discretion when working within the hospital.

3.5 TYPES OF INFUSION PUMPS AND DEVICES

3.5.1 Descriptions

(1) *Gravity infusion devices*

Gravity infusion devices, as their name implies, depend entirely on gravity to drive the infusion. They comprise an administration set containing a drip chamber and use a roller clamp to control the flow which is measured by counting drops. These have been in use for very many years and are suitable for infusing replacement fluids such as simple electrolytes which do not have to be infused with any particular degree of accuracy. The pressure developed for infusion depends entirely on the height of the liquid level in the container above the infusion site; at about one metre, the pressure is 70 mm Hg. The pressure in an adult peripheral vein is about 25 mm Hg so provided there is not too much resistance to flow through the cannula, the infusion will be satisfactory.

There are problems with maintaining an accurate flow - over a period of time, the tubing distorts and flattens within the roller clamp. The position of the clamp can also be disturbed. Both effects gradually reduce the rate of flow. Also, if there are high fluctuations in venous pressure, the flow can be reduced considerably.

The advantages of the gravity infusion device, also called *the gravity drip* or *standard solution set*, are the simplicity to set up and use, low cost, minimal risk of extravasation following an occlusion and minimal risk of introduction of air into the patient. The disadvantages are that the set cannot be used when resistance to flow is high. So infusions of viscous liquids are not possible. The device also needs frequent adjustment to keep the flow rate constant.

(2) *Common types of infusion pumps*

■ VOLUMETRIC PUMPS

These pumps administer large volume infusions and the rate is set directly in millilitres per hour. The accuracy of flow over an hour or more is usually well within 5 % which is more than adequate for the vast majority of clinical applications. Most volumetric pumps in use today employ the linear peristaltic mechanism which operates on straight tubing. A few do not but the mechanisms have similar accuracies. Volumetric pumps have many advantages: volumetric flow rates are delivered accurately, comprehensive alarm systems, e.g. to detect air in the administration set, an empty fluid bag and the occlusion pressure alarm setting. They can be used for both venous and arterial infusions, secondary infusions can often be delivered. The pumps have a Keep-vein-open (KVO) facility and some types directly measure the delivery pressure. However, volumetric pumps can be complicated to set up. All need a specific administration set and all pumps must be configured *only* to accept sets that are recommended by the manufacturers. The KVO facility reduces the administration rate after the end of the infusion so that the vein is kept patent.

■ SYRINGE PUMPS

Syringe pumps, as their name suggests, are devices that empty a syringe at a controlled rate. They are used extensively in High Dependency and Intensive Care Units where small volumes of highly concentrated drugs are delivered at low flow rates. They deliver smooth and accurate volumetric rates (millilitres per hour) and are easy to use. The pumps have a Keep-vein-open (KVO) facility and some types directly measure the delivery pressure. However, they suffer from some mechanical backlash although backlash can be compensated for in some newer models. Only the newer models have proper safeguards to prevent the syringe being fitted incorrectly and so guard against free flow.

Syringe pumps are used to administer drugs in concentrated solution for two reasons:

(1) Where fluid balance is important.
(2) When several drugs are needed that interact with one another. A multi-lumen in a central venous site is usually used in the ITU. Each drug enters the vein separately from the others by its own lumen and the rapid blood flow dilutes the drugs to prevent harmful interactions. If a peripheral infusion site is used, then the syringe pumps deliver the drugs via a 'Y' connector or a '3-way port' into the administration line which transports the fluid/diluent to the patient.

(3) Specialist types of infusion pumps

■ PATIENT CONTROLLED ANALGESIA (PCA) PUMPS

These enable a patient to self-administer a bolus of pain killing drug. Some are specialised volumetric and others are specialised syringe pumps. All designs have systems to prevent self-overdosing and several allow a constant background infusion to be automatically delivered.

■ ANAESTHESIA PUMPS

These are syringe pumps that have been specifically designed for the administration of anaesthetic agents and are *unsuitable* for any other use. They should only be used by anaesthetists.

■ AMBULATORY PUMPS

Ambulatory pumps are battery driven because they are carried around by the patient, whether at home or at the hospital. They are miniature versions of volumetric and syringe pumps and deliver the drug in a continual sequence of micro-boluses to conserve the battery. The term 'syringe driver' has been given to the ambulatory syringe pump.

■ OTHER DEVICES

There are several other types of non-electrically powered infusion devices that have no controls to set. These are fixed rate devices usually powered by an elastomeric membrane that has been stretched when loaded with a drug under pressure. The administration line, which is part of the device, contains a capillary tube that regulates flow on the assumption that the membrane returns to its original shape in a linear manner. These devices are often used for pain relief at home.

3.5.2 Risk classification of infusion pumps

The UK Department of Health classifies the suitability of ward-based infusion pumps for administering infusions of different degrees of risk. However, the system of classification has yet to be adapted to assess ambulatory devices. The Department regulates the designed performance of a pump so as to limit IV therapeutic risk. There are four categories of infusion risk:

(a) Neonatal risk infusions
(b) High risk infusions
(c) Lower risk infusions
(d) Ambulatory infusions.

(a) **Pumps suitable for neonatal infusions**

The first category, for neonatal infusions assumes that all infusions given by such pumps are high risk. The equipment therefore requires high accuracy and consistency of flow with 0.1 ml/hour increments, low occlusion alarm times and very low bolus on release of occlusion. In general, neonatal pumps have a wider range of features than are required in a low risk application and probably would not have the range of flow rates that are suitable for infusion into adults. Comprehensive alarm displays which identify the precise problem and safety interlocks to prevent tampering while running are important.

(b) **Pumps suitable for high risk infusions**

The second category, for high risk infusions, covers the infusion of drugs such as cardiac amines and oncological treatment drugs. This group requires high accuracy and consistency of flow, good occlusion alarm response, comprehensive alarm displays which identify the precise problem and safety interlocks.

Both neonatal and high risk pumps should have internal rechargeable battery back-up with a memory of parameters displayed so that vital data are not lost due to inadvertent switch off.

(c) **Pumps suitable for lower risk infusions**

The third category, for lower risk infusions, covers the infusion of simple electrolytes, antibiotics and total parenteral nutrition etc. The equipment does not need to be so accurate and consistent in output and need have only rudimentary alarm and safety systems. Battery back-up is not essential.

(d) **Pumps suitable for ambulatory infusions**

The fourth category, for ambulatory infusions, covers all infusion equipment which may be worn on the person so that normal activities can be continued while the infusion is being given. The equipment is often battery powered but clockwork mechanisms, elastomeric membranes or gas powered devices are also used.

3.5.3   Accuracy of infusion delivery

Neonatal and high risk infusion pumps must be accurate to within plus or minus 5% of the set rate when measured over a 60 minute period. They must also satisfy short term minute to minute requirements which determine smoothness and consistency of output. Pumps which suck back during infusion and have significant periods of zero flow cannot be used. Large fluctuations in delivered output are not permitted.

Pump performance requirements in terms of pressure, occlusion alarm delay time, size of bolus, etc. are listed in the publications of the UK Medical Devices Agency.

3.5.4 Matching pump to need

Choosing a pump means matching its performance to the needs of the infusion. Figures 9 and 10 show examples of real outputs from a syringe and a volumetric pump at 1 ml/hour. Mechanical backlash causes the syringe pump to take close to 40 minutes to achieve the set rate, this time being determined by the combination of the pump, the syringe and the rate. The flow pattern delivered by the volumetric pump is very different. The variations in flow rate are much larger than those of the syringe pump. The underlying regularity of volumetric pump output is caused by the repetition of the peristaltic pumping action.

Trumpet curves (Figures 11 and 12) are the way these variable outputs can be related to the needs of the infusion. The curves give the maximum over or under-infusion rate for any time interval in the infusion, from 1 to 35 minutes. Figures 11 and 12 are trumpet curves for a volumetric pump for two administration rates. For instance, short term variations in the delivery of fluids are not important providing that the patient receives the right amount over a long period of time. So a volumetric pump that is very inaccurate in the short term is suitable for delivery if it is accurate over the long term.

However, Figures 11 and 12 show that an inotrope, which has a half life of perhaps two minutes, will be subject to a maximum over- or under-infusion rate of 3% to 6% over intervals of two minutes. These variations may be large enough to allow significant changes in the accumulated dose received by the patient and so interfere with the stabilising action of the drug. A pump that has this level of short term inaccuracy may not be suitable for administering inotropes with very short half lives.

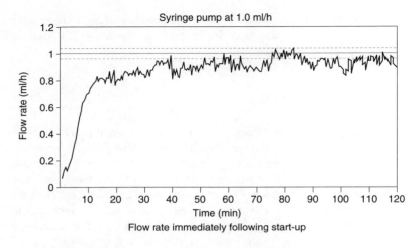

Fig. 9 Real output from a syringe pump at 1 ml per hour

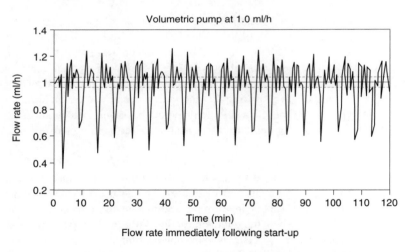

Fig. 10 Real output from a volumetric pump at 1 ml per hour

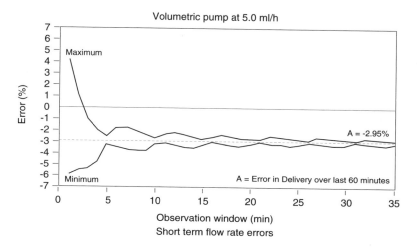

Fig. 11 Trumpet curve for a volumetric pump at 5 ml per hour

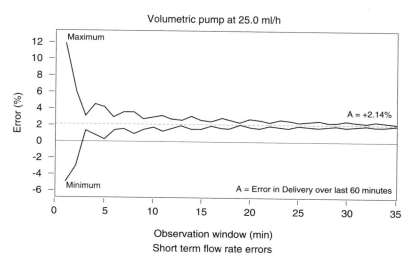

Fig. 12 Trumpet curve for a volumetric pump at 25 ml per hour

3.6 REVISION QUESTIONS

(1) State TWO reasons why a drug should not be administered as a concentrated solution.

(2) A drug has a long half-life (more than 48 hours). Using the half-life to guide your decision, state how the drug should be administered - by bolus or by infusion?

(3) What is the purpose of the needle inside a cannula?

(4) Why and for what type of infusion would there be a silicone insert in ordinary PVC tubing?

(5) What can cause air to be released from an infusate? Is this hazardous?

(6) How might free flow occur (a) from a gravity infusion device, (b) from a volumetric pump?

(7) Explain how siphonage from a syringe can occur.

(8) What factors would you need to consider when choosing an occlusion alarm pressure?

(9) What is mechanical backlash and what kinds of pumps exhibit it?

Answers to Revision Questions

Chapter 1

(1) 15% w/v
(2) 20% w/v
(3) 450 g/l
(4) 0.7%
(5) 25 g per 500 ml
(6) 2 ml
(7) 4 ml
(8) 1.5 ml/min; 90 ml/hour
(9) 120 ml/hour
(10) 0.24 ml/min; 14.4 ml/hour
(11) 1.6 ml/min and 96 ml/hour
(12) 51 drops/min and 3,060 drops/hour
(13) 24 drops/min
(14) The number of drops delivered by the set – see outer packaging.
(15) 1.04 ml/min; 62.5 ml/hour
(16) 22.64 mg

Chapter 2

(1) Hydrolysis, oxidation/reduction, photodegradation.
(2) Changing pH, dilution of a poorly soluble drug.
(3) Nitroprusside, Frusemide, Ergotamine, Vitamins A and K, Dacarbazine.
(4) Vitamins A, K, amphotericin B, frusemide, ergotamine, dacarbazine.
(5) Ensure correct pH.
(6) Poorly soluble - might overcome effect of any co-solvent.
(7) Changing pH and precipitation, drug-drug co-precipitation.
(8) If precipitation is suspected.
(9) Onto, into and through the plastic.
(10) PVC.
(11) Polyethylene.
(12) Minimize the risk of adsorption.
(13) (i)   Insulin, interferons
     (ii) Chlorpromazine diazepam, nimodipine, carmustine
     (iii) Nitrates, chlormethiazole, GTN/ISDN.
(14) Oxidation.
(15) Precipitation due to formation of an insoluble salt.

Chapter 3

(1) To avoid toxicity
     To avoid thrombophlebitis.
(2) Bolus.
(3) To puncture the vein and allow the cannula to enter the vein.
(4) To improve the accuracy of the administration rate of an infusion pump that uses the peristaltic pumping mechanism.
(5) Mechanical agitation of the fluid by volumetric pump mechanisms and the presence of nucleation sites. Hazardous to people with intracardiac circulation and to neonates.
(6) (a) Roller clamp open
     (b) Removal of the giving set from a volumetric pump with the roller clamp still open. The absence of an anti-free flow device in the set.
(7) (a) By gravity when the syringe is free to empty and at a height so that the head of fluid overcomes venous pressure, the friction in the plunger and the pressure drop in the administration line.
     (b) Air leakage into the syringe.
(8) The patient - neonate or adult.
     The drug prescribed.
     Resistance to flow in the administration set, filter and cannula or catheter.
     The drug administration rate.
(9) The delay between starting a syringe pump and the prescribed administration rate being achieved. Mechanical backlash is a feature of syringe pumps alone.

FURTHER READING LIST

Further Reading for Chapter 1

RE Anderson, JD Gatford. *Nursing Calculations*. Edinburgh: Churchill Livingstone, 1998.
JC LaRocca, SE Otto. *Pocket Guide to Intravenous Therapy*. St Louis: Mosby – Year Book Inc, 1997.
SJ Ogden, AG Opsahl. *Calculation of Drug Dosages*. St Louis: Mosby – Year Book Inc, 1991.

Further Reading for Chapter 2

For the topics of hydrolysis and oxidation/reduction:
P Mathews. *Advanced Chemistry 1 – Physical and Industrial*. Cambridge: Cambridge University Press, 1996.
R Lewis, W Evans. *Chemistry*. Basingstoke: Macmillan, 1997.

For the topics of acid/base equilibria, pH and solubility product:
GF Liptrot, JJ Thompson, GR Walker. *Modern Physical Chemistry*. London: Collins Educational, 1992.
EN Ramsden. *A - Level Chemistry*. Cheltenham: Stanley Thornes, 1994.

Further Reading for Chapter 3

Infusion Systems. MDA DB 9503. London: Medical Devices Agency, May 1995.
Syringe infusion pumps – review issue. *Evaluation* 1996; **283:** 1 – 88.
Volumetric infusion pumps – review issue. *Evaluation* 1996; **266:** 1 – 84.
Evaluation: Ambulatory Infusion Pumps. *Health Devices* 1991: **20(9):** 324 – 358.
Selection and Use of Infusion Devices for Ambulatory Applications. MDA DB 9703. London: Medical Devices Agency, March 1997.
Morling S. Infusion devices: risks and user responsibilities. *Br J Nursing* 1998; **7(1):** 13 – 20.
Pickstone M, Jacklin A, Auty B *et al*. Risk factors in IV infusions (Supplement). *Br J Int Care* 1995; **5(2):** 1 – 30.
Electromagnetic Compatibility of Medical Devices with Mobile Communications. MDA DB 9702. London: Medical Devices Agency, March 1997.
Richardson NH, Pickstone M. Interference from mobil phones in the ICU. *Br J Int Care* 1995; **5(7):** 233 – 235.
Electromagnetic Interference and Medical Devices. *Health Devices* 1996; **25(2-3):** 101 – 106.

MAIN INDEX

INDEX OF DRUGS